Farès Azaiez

Structured observation summary

Farès Azaiez

Structured observation summary

Pedagogical value in directed cardiology teaching

ScienciaScripts

Imprint

Cover image: www.ingimage.com

This book is a translation from the original published under ISBN 978-620-6-72487-2.

Publisher:
Sciencia Scripts
is a trademark of
Dodo Books Indian Ocean Ltd. and OmniScriptum S.R.L publishing group

120 High Road, East Finchley, London, N2 9ED, United Kingdom
Str. Armeneasca 28/1, office 1, Chisinau MD-2012, Republic of Moldova, Europe
Printed at: see last page
ISBN: 978-620-8-18815-3

TABLE OF CONTENTS

INTRODUCTION

Medical training requires the production of teaching resources that encourage students to actively acquire knowledge [1].

To achieve the objectives of this training, it is essential to choose the right learning method. There are several, each with its own characteristics and qualities. However, they are all based on the principle of reflection, enabling learners to become actively involved [2].

Among these means of learning in the field, directed teaching (DE) with the preparation of a structured summary of an observation (SSO) represents an original teaching method, based on contextualised learning and teaching based on cases. Complementing clinical placements, these OSR sessions aim to help students develop their clinical reasoning in terms of both general strategies and specific knowledge [2, 3].

The OSR session is geared towards solving a common pathology problem by drawing on prior knowledge, thereby facilitating the clinical reasoning process.

In addition, the OSR is not only a method of active learning but also a means of continuous formative assessment through the correction of these written observations [2].

To date, this DE has not been evaluated in cardiology training.

The aim of our study was to evaluate the interest of case-based DE by RSO in the learning of clinical reasoning in cardiology in first-year students of the second cycle of medical studies (DCEM1) at the Faculty of Medicine of Tunis (FMT).

METHODS

1 - Type of study

This was a descriptive monocentric cross-sectional study, carried out over the period from 17 January 2022 to 08 May 2022, on the evaluation of learning through directed teaching based on a real case in cardiology in the field, through the development of OSRs. This course was of interest to medical students assigned to a cardiology placement in the cardiology department of the Mongi Slim La Marsa Hospital during the second semester of the 2021/2022 academic year. It took place in the staff room of the same department.

2 - Population studied

We included in the study three groups of medical students in DCEM1 designated by the FMT internship department to each carry out a 5-week internship in the cardiology department of the Mongi Slim La Marsa Hospital during the study period. There were 9 to 11 students per group.

- Group 1: DCEM1 students affected by the FMT during the period from 17 January to 20 February 2022.
- Group 2: DCEM1 students assigned by the FMT during the period from 21 February to 03 April 2022.
- Group 3: DCEM1 students affected by the FMT during the period of 04 April to 08 May 2022.

This study did not include DCEM1 students who were absent from OSR development sessions.

3- Methodology

3- 1- Themes for directed teaching sessions:

Three sessions covering three different themes were held for each group.

The choice of theme was based on its frequency and/or urgency.

The pathologies chosen were included in the FMT medical curriculum.

They complied with the list of common and/or urgent pathologies in the cardiology training booklet (Appendix 1):

- Acute coronary syndrome (Theme 1)
- Acute lung oedema (Theme 2)
- Atrioventricular block (Theme 3)

3- 2- Planning sessions

Before the session took place, all the stages were planned in advance:

- The selection of clinical files relating to the themes chosen from the department's archives. These files included the patient's clinical, biological, echocardiographic, radiological, therapeutic and developmental data.

Photocopies of all the clinical observation documents were made according to the number of students in each session.

- A pre-test was carried out for each theme. It was identical for all three groups. It consisted of 5 multiple-choice questions (MCQs). The same pre-test was used as a post-test.

- The preparation of a satisfaction questionnaire with an evaluation based on the Likert scale. This questionnaire was used to evaluate the teaching provided.

- Announcing to students in advance the theme to be covered, inviting them to consult the self-teaching mini-module taught at the FMT corresponding to each theme.

- Explanation to students of the principle and stages of the session, including how this teaching method is to be assessed.

- Agreeing the date for the learning session with the students.

3- 3- Conduct of the session:

The session was scheduled to last between 60 and 75 minutes. It took place in the following stages:

- Welcome students and introduce the session.

- Completion of the pre-test (10 minutes). The mark awarded was out of 20. There was no minimum mark set for participation in the DE session.

- Distribution to each student of the clinical observation and the "Structured observation summary" form (Appendix 2).

- Students completed the various sections of the form (20 minutes). The work was done individually.

- Correct the observation in plenary, section by section, taking care to involve all the students, guide them, facilitate their progress through the stages, encourage discussion between them and manage the time (30 minutes).

- Decontextualisation of the pathology studied, taking into account the clinical, therapeutic and developmental particularities of the case.

- Post-test (5 minutes).

- Correction of the test in plenary.

- Completion of satisfaction questionnaire for session evaluation.

3- 4- Correction of the structured observation summary sheet

In addition to the student and patient identification sections, the form contains 16 sections for the learner to complete.

The grid was evaluated as follows:

- 0 wrong answer or no answer
- 0.5 correct answer incomplete
- 1 correct answer complete

The total score was based on 16 points.

Scores were considered good if between [12 and 16], average if between [8 and 12[and poor if below 8.

3- 5- Assessment of learning by the teacher

The pre-test scores were compared with the post-test scores. The percentage improvement in the pre-test averages compared with the post-test averages was compared using the following formula [4] :

(Average post-test - average pre-test) / average pre-test * 100

Improvement was considered satisfactory if the percentage was ≥ 10%.

3- 6- Teaching assessment

A satisfaction questionnaire was completed by the students at the end of each session in order to evaluate the teaching provided and to collect any difficulties perceived by the students and their perception of the contribution of this exercise to their learning.

It covered the following items:

- Assessment of the overall progress of the apprenticeship,
- Appreciation of the space and time allocated to learning,
- Clear objectives,
- Relevance of the subject,
- Active participation,
- Improving the clinical reasoning process.

This assessment was based on a Likert scale:

- Strongly disagree: - 2

- Somewhat disagree: - 1

- Somewhat agree: + 1

- Totally agree: + 2

4- Statistical analysis

The data were entered and analysed using EXCEL and SPSS 23 software for each of the three groups of students.

We carried out a descriptive study in which the qualitative variables were presented in numbers and percentages, and the quantitative variables in means and medians.

Comparisons of 2 means on paired series were made using the non-parametric Wilcoxon test for paired series. The significance level was set at 0.05.

5- Ethical considerations

The use of the test sheets, satisfaction and evaluation questionnaires and their exploitation in the context of a scientific project was announced to the students who consented.

The anonymity of the students was respected.

There was no conflict of interest in carrying out this work.

6- Bibliographical research

The bibliographic search was carried out using search engines such as "PubMed" and "Science direct" and at the FMT library using the following keywords:

Medical pedagogy, learning, clinical reasoning.

7- Writing the dissertation

We have followed the IMRAD format for scientific writing.

RESULTS

During the study period, nine DE sessions were given, three for each group. The same themes were covered in the three sessions provided for each group. These themes, as previously announced, were distributed as follows:

- Theme 1: Acute coronary syndrome

- Topic 2: Acute lung oedema

- Topic 3: Atrioventricular block

1- General characteristics of the sample

Of the 36 students assigned to the department during the study period, 31 (86%) attended OSR sessions.

1er group: 12 students: 11 present and 1 absent

2ème group: 13 students: 11 present and 2 absent

3ème group: 11 students: 9 present and 2 absent

Ninety-three OSRs were completed, i.e. 86% of the planned number (n=108).

2- Formative assessment of learners by the teacher

2-1- Overall and session-by-session assessment of RSO

The worksheets were marked for each session. The marks awarded to the sheets ranged from 5 to 15 for a total of 16 points. These marks were considered average in most cases, i.e. 60 OSRs (65%) (Table I).

Table I: Breakdown of RSO scores by session

	Session 1			Session 2			Session 3		
Notes	Poor	Means.	Good.	Poor	Means.	Good.	Poor	Means.	Good.
G1	3	8	0	2	7	2	1	7	3
G2	1	9	1	2	7	2	1	6	4
G3	3	5	1	1	6	2	1	5	3
Total	7	22	2	5	20	6	3	18	10

Good: Good, Poor: Poor, Avg. Average

We also noted an improvement in grade averages over the sessions, with the average rising from 9.12 to 11.92.

2-2- Evaluation of the different sections of the structured observation summary form

We have noted the difficulties encountered by learners when answering the different sections of the worksheet.

Group 1 (Table II) :

In all the sessions in the 1er group, the majority of students found no difficulty in answering the main problem, the reason for consultation and the reason for hospitalisation.

However, difficulties have been encountered concerning the data from non-specific paraclinical examinations in favour of a positive diagnosis, as well as the immediate and long-term prognosis.

In addition, the headings "Psychological state of this patient" and "Special features to report" were not completed throughout the three sessions.

Table II: Breakdown of correct answers to the "Structured observation summary" form by session and by heading for group 1

	Theme 1 (n=11)	Theme 2 (n=11)	Theme 3 (n=11)
Case study (the main problem)	8	9	9
Reasons for consultation	6	9	9
Reasons for hospitalisation	9	10	9
Anamnestic data in favour of a positive diagnosis of the main problem	3	7	7
Physical examination data in favour of a positive diagnosis of the main problem	6	5	6
Non-specific paraclinical data in favour of a positive diagnosis	2	2	3
Decisive arguments in favour of the diagnosis of the disease and its origin	4	6	5
Other diagnoses discussed and ruled out by appropriate tests carried out on this patient	2	3	6
Associated pathologies or anomalies	6	4	8
Psychological state of this patient	-	-	-

Immediate prognosis and arguments in favour	1	0	1
Treatment decisions	2	4	3
Evolution	1	3	7
Elements of remote prognosis	3	2	4
Treatment prescribed on discharge	2	5	3
Particularities to note about the disease	-	-	-

Group 2 (Table III) :

The main difficulties for the 2ème group concerned differential diagnoses.

In addition, the headings for "Psychological state of this patient" and "Special features to report" were not filled in equally throughout the three sessions.

Table III: Breakdown of complete correct answers on the "Structured observation summary" form by session and by heading for group 2

	Theme 1 (n=11)	**Theme 2 (n=11)**	**Theme 3 (n=11)**
Case study (the main problem)	7	9	7
Reasons for consultation	6	8	9
Reasons for hospitalisation	9	9	9
Anamnestic data in favour of a positive diagnosis of the main problem	3	5	6

Physical examination data in favour of a positive diagnosis of the main problem	4	6	6
Non-specific paraclinical data in favour of a positive diagnosis	5	2	7
Decisive arguments in favour of the diagnosis of the disease and its origin	4	6	8
Other diagnoses discussed and ruled out by appropriate tests carried out on this patient	2	1	2
Associated pathologies or anomalies	5	5	7
Psychological state of this patient	-	-	-
Immediate prognosis and arguments in favour	4	6	5
Treatment decisions	5	4	6
Evolution	5	3	8
Elements of remote prognosis	5	6	8
Treatment prescribed on discharge	4	4	6
Particularities to note about the disease	-	-	-

Group 3 (Table IV) :

The main difficulty for the students in the 3ème group concerned the anamnesis data in favour of a positive diagnosis of the main problem, where only 5 complete correct answers were collected at the end of the three sessions.

In addition, the headings "Psychological state of this patient" and "Particularities to report" were only completed by one student for each of the three sessions in group 3.

Table IV: Breakdown of complete correct answers on the "Structured observation summary" form by session and by heading for group 3

	Theme 1 (n=9)	Theme 2 (n=9)	Theme 3 (n=9)
Case study (the main problem)	4	8	7
Reasons for consultation	6	7	7
Reasons for hospitalisation	6	6	8
Anamnestic data in favour of a positive diagnosis of the main problem	1	2	2
Physical examination data in favour of a positive diagnosis of the main problem	6	5	7
Non-specific paraclinical data in favour of a positive diagnosis	3	6	6
Decisive arguments in favour of the diagnosis of the disease and its origin	4	5	5
Other diagnoses discussed and ruled out by appropriate tests carried out on this patient	4	3	4
Associated pathologies or anomalies	6	5	7
Psychological state of this patient	1	-	-
Immediate prognosis and arguments in favour	3	3	5

Treatment decisions	5	4	6
Evolution	2	3	7
Elements of remote prognosis	3	3	4
Treatment prescribed on discharge	4	5	3
Particularities to note about the disease	-	1	-

3- Assessment of teaching by the teacher :

All the students present took the pre-test. The average pre-test scores by group and topic are shown in Table IV.

Table IV: Breakdown of pre-test scores by session

	Theme 1	Theme 2	Theme 3
Group 1	12,2	13,1	13,4
Group 2	11,9	14,2	12,4
Group 3	12,7	13,1	13,7
Average	12,3	13,5	13,2

Post-test scores were generally higher than pre-test scores, as shown in Figure 1.

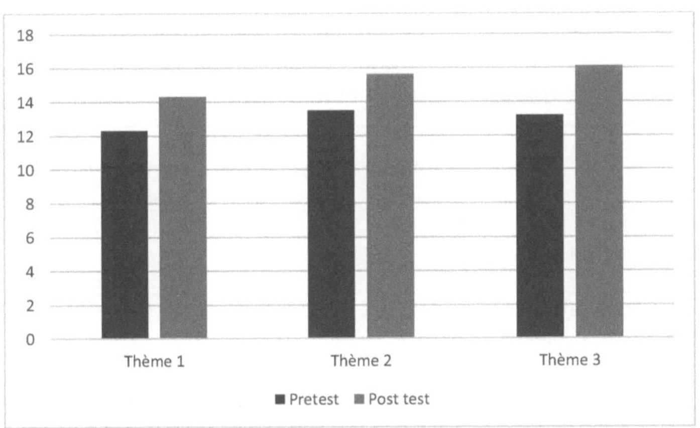

Figure 1: Trend in average test scores by theme

The improvement was statistically significant and satisfactory for all three themes, with p=0.001, p=0.003 and p=0.002 respectively.

IV- Evaluation of teaching by students

A total of 186 student responses to the satisfaction questionnaire were collated (Table V).

The majority of students (91%) were satisfied with the overall learning experience.

The time and/or space allocated to this learning was deemed satisfactory in 87% of cases.

Students felt that they participated actively during the learning sessions and that this teaching facilitated the process of their clinical reasoning (≥ 90%).

Table V: Students' overall assessment of teaching

	-2 I totally disagree	-1 Somewhat disagree	+1 Somewhat agree	+2 I totally agree
1- Assessment of the overall conduct of the session	1 (3%)	2 (6%)	9 (29%)	19 (62%)
2- Appreciation of the space and time allocated to learning	1 (3%)	3 (10%)	11 (35%)	16 (52%)
3- Clear objectives	0	4 (13%)	6 (19%)	21 (68%)
4- Relevance of the subject	0	1 (3%)	12 (39%)	18 (58%)
5- Active participation	0	2 (6%)	2 (6%)	27 (88%)
6- Improving clinical reasoning	0	3 (10%)	2 (6%)	26 (84%)

DISCUSSION

1- Main results of our study

We conducted a descriptive cross-sectional study from 17 January 2022 to 08 May 2022 in the cardiology department of the Mongi Slim Hospital, La Marsa, with the aim of evaluating the value of case-based DE by OSR in the learning of clinical reasoning in cardiology in FMT DCEM1 students.

A total of nine DE sessions involving 31 students were run and 93 OSR forms were completed.

The themes chosen were acute coronary syndrome (theme 1), acute pulmonary oedema (theme 2) and atrioventricular block (theme 3).

Once the OSR sheets had been corrected, it was noted that the average scores improved as the sessions progressed.

The main difficulties encountered by the students concerned the headings relating to "Psychological state of this patient" and "Special features to report", which were only completed on one form each.

By comparing the test scores before (pre-test) and at the end of the session (post-test), a statistically significant improvement was noted for the 3 themes.

The response to the satisfaction questionnaire showed that the majority of students were satisfied with the overall learning process (91%). They felt that the teaching facilitated their clinical reasoning (90%).

2- Strengths and limitations of the study

➢ <u>Highlights of the study</u>

- Relevance of the subject: this study assessed the value of OSR as a means of learning in the cardiology training field.
- The relatively large number of OSRs obtained made it possible to carry out a statistical study and to highlight the significance of the learners' development through this teaching.
- This study assessed the applicability of the OSR form in cardiology. Some sections were not completed. Changes need to be made to make the form easier to understand and use.

➢ <u>Limitations of the study :</u>

- The limits of pre-testing :

Only five MCQs were given to the students for the pre-tests, whereas Dr Tabbane, in the chapter entitled "Travaux dirigés en stage d'externat" ("Tutorials during the clerkship") in his book "Eléments d'introduction aux ateliers de pédagogie médicale" ("Elements of an introduction to medical teaching workshops"), suggests giving around twenty true-false type items [1]. In order to respect the time allocated to the session, we were unable to ask as many questions during the pre-test.

- Heterogeneous student involvement during the sessions
- The limits of post-testing :

Carried out directly at the end of the session, it only allows us to explore the student's short-term memory and not the impact of the new knowledge on practice or on long-term changes in behaviour.

3- Active case-based learning methods:

Transmissive teaching methods are tending to disappear, to be replaced by active teaching methods in which the student is at the centre of his or her own learning [5, 6].

At their core, these active teaching methods aim to focus on the student's activity rather than that of the teacher.

Among active learning methods, the importance of observation-based teaching is well established [7].

This active engagement, a pillar of learning, fosters curiosity and autonomy [8]. It also increases the learner's level of motivation in relation to the tasks proposed.

This active learning is therefore based on an authentic and complex real-life situation that involves common scenarios aligned with learning objectives and that has the characteristic of being stimulating for learners.

Case-based learning is one of the learning strategies used in medical studies. Its main feature is that it uses real-life cases to better prepare students for clinical practice [9].

Other means of active case-based learning include :

- Learning to reason clinically (ARC)
- Problem-based learning (PBL) [10]
- Case Based Learning (CBL) [11].

4- Assessment of learning

Assessment of learning is an essential part of the teaching-learning process; it is necessary and part of teaching [12].

Kirkpatrick's 4-level evaluation model dates back to 1959 and is the most widely used by those interested in training evaluation (Figure 2); it summarises the complex evaluation process and simplifies it [13].

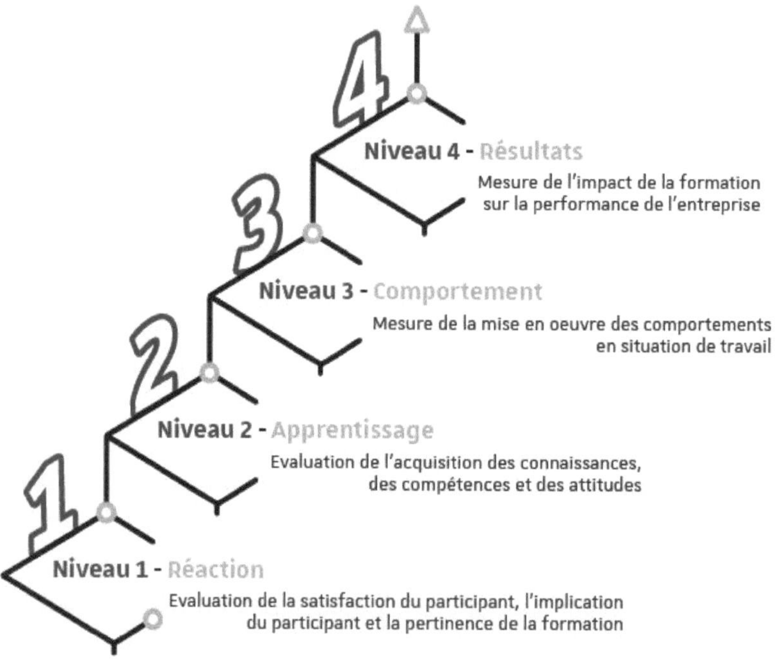

Figure 2: The Kirkpatrick model

In our case, it is a formative assessment concerning Kirkpatrick's level 2, i.e. the assessment of the student's learning and acquisition of knowledge.

In fact, the learning process used in our study, the OSR, also forms part of a formative assessment of learners, through the teacher's marking of learners' answers to the various headings.

5- Assessment of teaching

➢ Teacher assessment of teaching :

This teaching enables teachers to assess the quality and level of their teaching and, if necessary, to modify the content or methods [14].

In our study, the statistically significant improvement in test averages at the end of the sessions for the different themes simply reflects the progress of the learning process.

➢ Evaluation of teaching by learners :

To evaluate the teaching by the learners, we used a questionnaire at the end of each session, which enabled us to collect the students' assessments. This is an evaluation of student satisfaction (Kirkpatrick level 1).

The Likert scale was used for this evaluation. Six items were processed.

Feedback was positive. All the students confirmed that this method helped to improve their clinical reasoning. These favourable testimonies are in line with the results of international research [15, 16], as well as with previous Tunisian studies [9, 17].

6- The place of case-based teaching in the form of structured observation summaries in active learning

The OSR summarises the diagnostic approach in actual professional practice, including headings covering clinical and paraclinical aspects, positive diagnosis, aetiological diagnosis, differential diagnoses, short- and long-term prognosis, as well as the therapeutic approach and the course of the disease.

By filling in these sections, the learner repeats the diagnostic process, identifies gaps and selects only relevant information from the detailed summary of the observation.

This activity prepares students to produce structured and relevant summaries of clinical observations during their clinical placements.

Studying the medical file confronts students with a situation linked to their future professional context ("contextualisation" phase). They must be able to extract the principles of reasoning ("decontextualisation") and apply them to other situations. In this learning and reasoning process, the tutor plays a role in helping the student to become aware of his or her shortcomings and to integrate the data more effectively.

This teaching method, which is DE by RSO, can be considered as a variant of DE from a known case.

7- Outlook

Students' satisfaction with DE by RSO suggests that its scope of application should be extended to all placement sites. As a result, there is a need to intensify training and to introduce teachers, in particular placement supervisors, to this teaching method.

However, some changes seem necessary and should be made to this standard sheet.

The section on "Patient's psychological state" was not completed throughout the sessions due to a lack of data in the clinical records. Assessment of the patient's psychological state in all disciplines is fundamental. This study highlighted the gaps in our records.

The last section, "Particularities to report relating to the disease", was not completed throughout the sessions. This could be due to a lack of data or perhaps the irrelevance of this section.

CONCLUSIONS

The development of OSRs represents an original teaching method, based on contextualised learning and teaching from solved cases, developed and implemented in the FMT externship clinical placements.

The aim of our study was to evaluate the value of case-based DE by OSR in teaching clinical reasoning in cardiology to FMT DCEM1 students.

We conducted a descriptive cross-sectional study involving three groups of students assigned to the cardiology department of Mongi Slim La Marsa Hospital during the second semester of the 2021/2022 academic year.

During the study period, nine guided teaching sessions were carried out, i.e. three sessions per group. The same topics were covered in all three groups, namely acute coronary syndrome, acute pulmonary oedema and atrioventricular block.

The teacher's teaching was evaluated by marking the OSR sheets completed by the learners and by comparing the pre- and post-test scores.

The students' evaluation of the teaching was based on a satisfaction questionnaire.

Thirty-one students took part in the OSR sessions.

When the OSR sheets were corrected, the scores were mostly average (65%), with an improvement in scores over the sessions.

The main difficulties with the OSR form concerned the headings "Patient's psychological state" and "Particularities to report relating to the disease".

Post-test scores were significantly higher than pre-test scores.

The response to the satisfaction questionnaire showed that the majority of students were satisfied with the overall learning process (91%). They felt that the content of the sessions was relevant and that the teaching facilitated their clinical reasoning (90%).

Finally, although this active learning method does not cover many objectives, it is based on real contexts that are meaningful to the student, which can increase their level of motivation for the tasks proposed. In this way, it promotes sustainable learning.

This method should therefore be more widely used for placements in the various specialities.

REFERENCES

1- Langevin S, Hivon R. En quoi l'externat ne s'acquitte t- il pas adéquatement de son mandat pédagogique? A qualitative study based on a systematic analysis of the literature. Pédagogie Médicale. 2007;8(1):7-23.

2- Marrakchi J. Pedagogical interest of structured observation summaries in otorhinolaryngology. *Medicine: Tunis.* 2018

3- C Tabbane. Elements of introduction to medical pedagogy workshops. *Centre de Publication Universitaire.* 2000

4- How do I calculate the percentage increase or reduction in Excel? [Online]. Your Assistant [14/01/2015]. http:// www.votreassistante.net

5- Presseau A, Frenay M. Le transfert des apprentissages. Québec: Presses de l'Université Laval; 2004. p7

6- Bédard D, Frenay M, Turgeon J, Paquay L. Les fondements de dispositifs pédagogiques visant à favoriser le transfert de connaissances: perspectives de l'apprentissage et de l'enseignement. Res Academica. 2000;18:21-47.

7- Vanpee D. What the perspective of authentic contextualised learning and teaching can contribute to optimising the pedagogical quality of clerkships. Pédagogie Médicale. 2010;10:253-66.

8- Dehaene S. Learning! The talent of brains, the challenge of machines. Odile Jacob; 2018.

9- Ben Neji H. Directed teaching based on real observations in clinical haematology. [Dissertation]. Medicine: Tunis; 2018.26p.

10- Srinivasan M, Wilkes M, Stevenson F, Nguyen T, Slavin S. Comparing problem-based learning with case-based learning: effects of a major curricular shift at two institutions. Academic medicine. 2007;82(1):74-82.

11- Williams B. Case based learning a review of the literature: is there scope for this educational paradigm in prehospital education? EMJ. 2005;22(8):577-81.

12- Jouquan J. L'évaluation des apprentissages des étudiants en formation médicale. Pédagogie médicale. 2002;3(1):38-52.

13- Yardley S, Dorman T. Kirkpatrick's levels and education evidence. Med Educ. 2012;46:97-106.

14- Gilibert D, Gillet I. Review of training evaluation models: individual and social conceptual approaches. Prat Psychol. 2010;16(3):217-38.

15- Zahng SY, Zheng JW, Yang C, Zhang ZY, Shen GF, Zahng JZ, et al. Case-based learning in clinical courses in a Chinese college of stomatology. Journal of dental education. 2012;76(10):1389-92.

16- Mackenzie CT. Dental student perceptions of case-based educational effectiveness. Journal of dental education. 2013;77(6):688-93.

17- Zehani A. Intérêt pédagogique de l'enseignement dirigé en Anatomie Pathologique pour la formation médicale. [Mémoire]. Médecine : Tunis; 2018.23p.

APPENDICES

APPENDIX 1: DCEM1 clinical placement logbook (FMT)

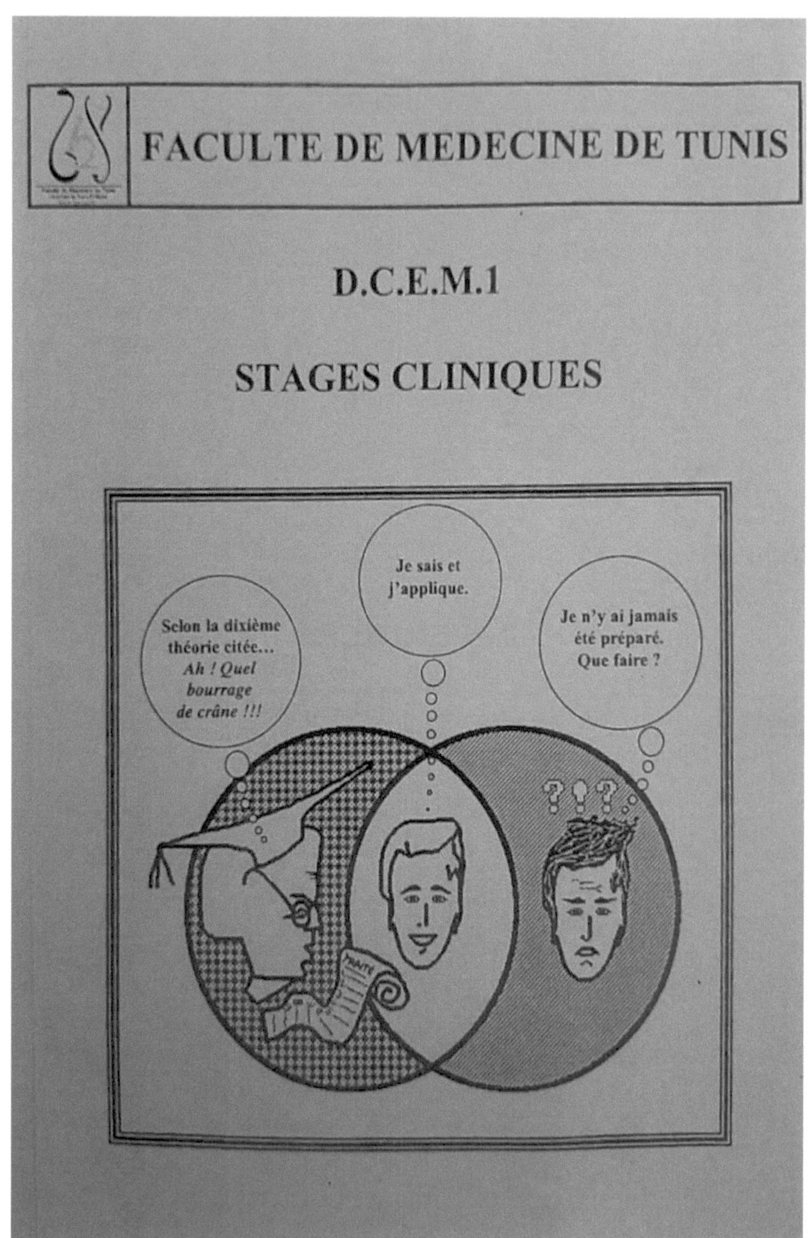

OBJECTIFS ET EVALUATION DU STAGE DE PATHOLOGIE CARDIOVASCULAIRE

OBJECTIFS[1]	Enseigné[2]	Evalué[3]	
		Note	Signature
Objectifs relatifs à l'habileté technique :			
1.Procéder à une anamnèse objective, complète et précise en se référant au formulaire ou au protocole d'interrogatoire en usage dans le service. En vue notamment de :			
-Recueillir les caractéristiques d'une douleur thoracique et distinguer un angor d'une autre douleur thoracique, en le décrivant selon la classification canadienne ;			
-Classer une dyspnée en stade NYHA, et reconnaitre les caractéristiques d'une dyspnée d'origine cardiaque ;			
-Reconnaitre des palpitations, une syncope et en préciser les caractéristiques.			
2. Pratiquer l'examen physique méthodique et complet en vue de :			
2.1.Reconnaître à l'inspection une dyspnée, une cyanose, une turgescence des jugulaires ;			
2.2.Palper la région précordiale : -pour y localiser le choc de pointe ; -pour rechercher un frémissement, un signe de Harzer ;			
2.3.Localiser les 4 principaux foyers d'auscultation cardiaque ;			
2.4. Ausculter le cœur en vue de : *Utiliser des méthodes audio-visuelles pour compléter l'apprentissage si nécessaire.*			
-déterminer le rythme et la fréquence cardiaque ;			
-reconnaître : . le 1er bruit et le 2ème bruit ; . un éclat ou un dédoublement de B1 ou B2 (en préciser le foyer) ; . un rythme en 3 temps ; un galop proto ou télédiastolique			
-identifier un souffle ou un roulement éventuel et en décrire le siège, le temps, l'intensité, le timbre et les irradiations ;			
-identifier un autre bruit surajouté : frottement péricardique, claquement d'ouverture mitral, click ;			
-reconnaitre des bruits de prothèse valvulaire mécanique.			
2.5.Percuter et ausculter les aires pleuro-pulmonaires à la recherche d'une matité, de râles crépitants ;			
2.6.Rechercher une hépatomégalie et un reflux hépatojugulaire ;			
2.7.Mesurer la pression artérielle (PA) de façon bilatérale, en décubitus et en orthostatisme ;			

[1] A réaliser en situation réelle ou simulée (R ou S).
[2] C'est-à-dire, a fait l'objet d'une démonstration pratique (colonne à remplir par l'étudiant). Inscrire R ou S (ou 0 si pas de démonstration).
[3] A fait l'objet d'un ou plusieurs contrôle(s) dont seul le dernier a donné lieu à la note définitive inscrite et attestée par une signature. Inscrire NE si non évalué.

DCEM1 (31)

OBJECTIFS[1]	Enseigné[2]	Evalué[3]	
		Note	Signature
2.8. Procéder à Un examen vasculaire bilatéral et comparatif comprenant (outre la mesure de la PA) : - une palpation des pouls, - une auscultation des axes artériels, - une identification et localisation de varices, - un test d'Allen, - un index de pression systolique (cheville/bras) ;			
2.9. Rechercher des signes de phlébite (membre inférieur chaud, oedématié, douloureux, signe de Homans) ;			
2.10. Procéder à un examen périphérique à la recherche : - d'œdèmes des membres inférieurs (distinguer les œdèmes de type rénal des autres types d'œdèmes), - des troubles trophiques en rapport avec une insuffisance artérielle ou veineuse ;			
2.11. Regrouper les signes cliniques élémentaires en syndromes aigus ou chroniques (dont les syndromes d'insuffisance coronaire et d'insuffisance cardiaque gauche, droite et globale).			
3. Consigner les données cliniques.			
4. Interpréter les examens paracliniques suivants :			
4.1. Réaliser une lecture méthodique d'un électrocardiogramme en vue de :			
-vérifier l'identification, les caractéristiques et la qualité de l'enregistrement ; -repérer P, QRS, T, PR, ST et QT, et reconnaître leurs variations physiologiques et pathologiques ; -déterminer l'axe de QRS ;			
-reconnaître : . une anomalie de rythme ou de fréquence cardiaque, . un bloc de conduction sino-atrial ou auriculo-ventriculaire et un bloc de branche, . une pré-excitation ventriculaire, . un allongement du QT, . un trouble de l'excitabilité supra-ventriculaire ou ventriculaire, . des signes d'ischémie ou de nécrose myocardique, . des signes d'hypertrophie cavitaire droite ou gauche, . des signes de péricardite, . un rythme électro-entraîné (stimulation cardiaque).			
4.2. Radiographies standards de thorax pour :			
-reconnaître les différents arcs de la silhouette cardiaque avec leurs variations pathologiques ;			
-mesurer le rapport cardiothoracique ;			
-apprécier la vascularisation pulmonaire ;			
-identifier un épanchement pleural.			

OBJECTIFS[1]	Enseigné[2]	Evalué[3]	
		Note	Signature
4.3. Autres examens complémentaires (Préciser leur indication, lire et utiliser les résultats) :			
-Dosages des marqueurs cardiaques ; -Imagerie cardiaque (Echographie cardiaque transthoracique et imagerie de coupe) ; -Epreuve d'effort et examens de stress ; -Coronarographie ; -Enregistrement ambulatoire de pression artérielle ; -Enregistrement ambulatoire de rythme cardiaque.			
5. Pratiquer les soins suivants :			
-Enregistrement d'un E.C.G. 17 dérivations.			
Objectifs relatifs à la solution des problèmes de santé[4] :			
6. Sur le plan diagnostic :		**Epreuve spécifique. cf. page 8 paragraphe 5.2.2.**	
6.1. Discuter le diagnostic différentiel chez l'adulte et chez l'enfant devant des manifestations cardiaques (hypertension artérielle, souffle cardiaque, cyanose, douleur thoracique, dyspnée aiguë, dyspnée chronique, palpitations...) selon une démarche appropriée.			
6.2. Suspecter ou reconnaître :			
-les cas simples de pathologie courante ;			
-les urgences les plus fréquentes.			
7. Participer à la **prise en charge** des affections courantes et des urgences, comprenant : l'évaluation du risque, le conditionnement et la mise en place des élements de surveillance, l'organisation d'un éventuel transfert et la prescription de traitement médicamenteux ou non pharmacologique.			
Objectifs relatifs aux attitudes :			
8.Manifester les attitudes décrites dans le chapitre 2.2. de la page 5.			

[4] Voir liste ci-après présentée à titre indicatif sous réserve de modification par le service où se déroule le stage.

PATHOLOGIES COURANTES :	URGENCES :
- Angor stable.	- Syndromes coronaires aigus.
- Hypertension artérielle.	- Péricardite aigue et tamponnade.
- Valvulopathies mitrale et aortique.	- Endocardites infectieuses.
- Cardiomyopathies dilatée et hypertrophique.	- Œdème aigu du poumon.
- Insuffisance cardiaque.	- Embolie pulmonaire.
- Fibrillation auriculaire.	- Blocs auriculo-ventriculaires.
- Artérite oblitérante des membres inférieurs.	- Tachycardies ventriculaires et supraventriculaires
	- Urgences hypertensives.
	- Ischémie aigue des membres inférieurs.
	- Troubles du rythme ventriculaire.

APPENDIX 2: Structured observation summary form

RESUME STRUCTURE D'OBSERVATION

Nom de l'externe :	Stage en :	Chef de service :
Cas étudiè *(précisez le problème principal)* :		
Prénom du patient : Numéro du dossier:	Age :	Originaire de : Demeurant à :
Entré le :	) Sorti ou DCD le :	

Motifs de consultation *(troubles, ancienneté, consultations médicales antérieures...)*	
Motifs d'hospitalisation	
Données d'anamnèse en faveur du diagnostic positif du problème principal *(facteurs prédisposant, déclenchant, constitutionnels, familiaux...)*	
Données d'examen physique en faveur du diagnostic positif du problème principal	
Données d'examens paracliniques non spécifiques en faveur du diagnostic positif *(examens de 1° intention)*	
Arguments décisifs en faveur du diagnostic de la maladie et de son origine *(argument ou ensemble d'arguments spécifique(s))*	
Autres diagnostics discutés et éliminés par des examens appropriés pratiqués chez ce patient	
Pathologies ou anomalies associées *(etat de nutrition, maladie chronique, allergie à un médicament, ...)*	
Etat psychologique de ce patient *(gaieté, tristesse, angoisse, réaction à la maladie ...)*	
Pronostic immédiat et arguments en faveur *(paramètres vitaux et autres arguments spécifiques...)*	
Décisions thérapeutiques *(abstention, nature du ou des traitements, durée du ou des traitements...)*	
Evolution *(délai de régression des signes cliniques et para-cliniques, signes persistants, complications liées à la maladie ou d'origine iatrogène...)*	
Eléments du pronostic éloigné *(risque de récidives ou de séquelles selon la maladie et les caractéristiques psychologique, socio-économique et culturelle)*	
Traitement prescrit à la sortie *(medicaments, traitement autre que médicamenteux, conseils prodigués...)*	
Particularités à signaler relatives à la maladie *(atypies : clinique, paraclinique, évolutive...)* associées *(autres pathologies, contexte particulier du patient...)*	

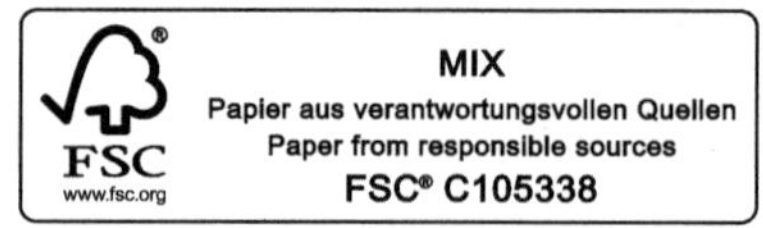

Printed by Books on Demand GmbH, Norderstedt / Germany